TABLE OF CONTENTS

INTRODUCTION

In the 39th year of King Asa's rule, he was diseased in his feet until his disease was very critical. Yet, in his disease, he did not seek the Lord, but went to the physicians for help. He died two years later. [2 Chronicles 16:11-13]

There is nothing wrong with going to physicians or seeking medical help or advice. But what we should do is seek the LORD first to see what he wants us to do. He may want to heal us by His sovereign power, over a period of time, or instantaneously.

- You must know that healing belongs to you. There is no need for you to depart from health.

- You can be healed and walk in health – and -- You can help others to do the same.

Baruch haba b'Shem Adonai

Prince Handley

Health and Healing

Complete Guide to Wholeness

~

Victory Over Sickness and Disease

The dictionary defines "disease" as: 1) any departure from a state of health; 2) a disordered condition of mind or body marked by definite symptoms.

To be at "ease" is to be FREE from pain or any discomfort, including anxiety and stress. "Dis-ease" is the opposite. In the Holy Bible, God promised MORE than healing for his people. He promised DIVINE HEALTH: freedom from disease!

5

"If you will carefully listen to the voice of the Lord your God, and will do that which is right in his sight, and will give ear to his commandments, and keep all his statutes, I will put none of these diseases upon you ... for I am the LORD that heals you." [Torah: Exodus 15:26]

Notice the last phrase: "I am the LORD that heals you." Literally, the Hebrew language is saying, "I am **Jehovah Rapha** (The LORD, your physician)." It is wonderful to be able to claim God's promises for divine healing, but it is even better to walk in divine HEALTH: not needing to be healed!

Exodus 23:25 says, "And you shall serve the LORD your God and he shall bless your bread, and your water; and I will take sickness away from the midst of you." When sickness is "away" from you, then you have HEALTH. Thank God, it is His will for **YOU** to walk in divine health just as much as it is for your soul to be saved. In 3 John, verse 2, (a passage of scripture which is written to Christians) the Holy Bible says:

"Beloved, I wish above all things that you may prosper AND BE IN HEALTH, even as your soul prospers."

Psalm 103 gives us a powerful promise from God to any and ALL who may be suffering from disease: spiritual, physical, or mental.

"Bless the LORD, O my soul: and all that is within me, bless his holy name.

Bless the LORD, O my soul, and forget not all his benefits:

Who forgives all your iniquities (or sins); who HEALS ALL YOUR DISEASES." [Psalm 103:1-3]

God's nature never changes. The same healing nature of God that was revealed in the Old Testament of the Holy Bible is revealed in the New Testament. His nature is the same today as it was yesterday. In the Old Testament, God said, "For I am the LORD, I change not." In the New Testament we read, "Jesus Christ the same yesterday, and today, and forever." [Malachi 3:6 and Hebrews 13:8]

Jesus displayed the healing nature of God, Jesus said, "He that has seen me has seen the Father." [John 14:9] Jesus never refused healing to anyone! Jesus' nature is God's nature. He never refused healing to anyone. Jesus is God!

"And Jesus went about all the cities and villages, teaching in their synagogues, and preaching the gospel [good news] of the kingdom, and healing EVERY disease among the people." [Matthew 9:35]

Jesus came to earth to heal - to restore to health: spiritually, physically, and mentally. He came to "buy" back what Adam, the first man who ever lived, lost. In the Garden of Eden, Adam sinned against God by disobeying him. God had commanded Adam:

"Of every tree of the garden you may freely eat. But of the tree of the knowledge of good and evil, you shall not eat of it; for in the day you shall eat of it you shall surely die." [Genesis 2:16-17]

Satan, the devil, lied to Eve, Adam's wife, saying, "You shall not surely die." But Eve, like many people today, did not realize that REAL death is "spiritual"! Physical death (when your body dies) is merely a **result** of "spiritual" death. To be spiritually dead does not mean you do not exist; it simply means you exist, but that you are SEPARATED from God: "joined" to Satan!

From one act of disobedience by Adam, sin entered into the world, so that spiritual death passed through the bloodline to ALL men ... resulting in physical death.

"Wherefore, as by one man [Adam] sin entered into the world, and death by sin; so death passed upon ALL men, for all have sinned." [Romans 5:12]

This "spiritual" death - SEPARATION FROM GOD - which produced physical sickness and disease, and the death of the body, HAD TO BE HEALED! This is why God sent his only Son, Jesus Christ, to earth.

"For as by one man's disobedience many were made sinners, so by the OBEDIENCE of one [Jesus Christ] shall many be made righteous." [Romans 5:19]

In Isaiah Chapter 53 we see just what Jesus did ... why he came to earth!

"Surely he has borne our sicknesses and diseases, and carried [away] our pains; yet we did esteem him stricken, smitten of God and afflicted. [Verse 4]

But he was wounded for our transgressions, he was bruised for our iniquities: the chastisement of our peace was upon him; AND WITH HIS STRIPES WE ARE HEALED. [Verse 5]

All we like sheep have gone astray; we have turned everyone to his own way, and the LORD has laid on him the iniquity [or, sin] of us all." [Verse 6]

What Isaiah prophesied in the Old Testament was fulfilled 750 years later by the Messiah of Israel, Yeshua Ha Mashiach [Jesus the "Christ", or the "Anointed One"]. He bore **our** sicknesses and diseases. He carried away **our** pains. He was wounded and bruised for **our** sin; the LORD laid on him the sin of us all. And with his stripes we are healed.

In some Bibles Isaiah 53:4 reads: "Surely he has borne our 'griefs' and carried our 'sorrows'." However, the original Hebrew (the original language of the Hebrew Scriptures) for the words "grief" and "sorrow" is "choli" and "macob", respectively. "Choli" means "sickness and disease". "Macob" means "pain" (acute pain; intense suffering: mental or physical).

To prove that Isaiah meant in this passage that healing would be included in Messiah's work for us, we need only to consult the New Testament record of Jesus' ministry in Matthew Chapter 8, verses 16-17:

"When the evening was come, they brought unto him many that were possessed with devils; and he cast out the spirits with his word, and healed ALL that were sick.

That it might be fulfilled which was spoken by Isaiah the prophet, saying, 'Himself [Jesus the Messiah] took our infirmities, and bore our sicknesses'."

Jesus fulfilled what Isaiah the prophet said 750 years before:

- He bore **our** sicknesses and diseases.
- He carried away **our** pains.
- With his stripes **WE ARE HEALED**.

Jesus' body and mind took punishment for **us** ... his blood paid for **our** sins. His body was beaten, wounded and bruised (even before he was crucified) and then he was nailed to the wooden cross ... FOR **OUR** HEALING: spiritual, physical, and mental!

Oppression - both mental and physical - is included in Christ's work for **us**. Christ was driven; he was abased and looked down upon. Isaiah 53:7 says, "He was oppressed and he was afflicted ..."

In Isaiah 53:4, where it reads, " … he carried our 'pains' …", the literal Hebrew meaning is "acute pain; intense suffering: MENTAL or PHYSICAL." What Jesus did FOR you, you don't have to do!

Jesus healed the separation between God and man through his work FOR US, and therefore ended Satan's dominion over ALL who would trust in Christ! "For this purpose the Son of God was manifested, that he might DESTROY the works of the devil." [1 John 3:8]

Jesus "carried" sickness, sin, disease, poverty, and oppression - the works of the devil (Satan) - FOR YOU. Now you don't have to carry them any longer. They do NOT belong to the believer in Christ!

WHAT JESUS DID FOR YOU …

YOU DON'T HAVE TO DO!

Now that you know that physical and mental healing belong to the believer in Christ - as much as spiritual healing - you need to know how to obtain it: HOW TO BE HEALED! There are several ways, or avenues, to obtain AND to minister Christ's healing power. They are listed below:

● THE WORD OF GOD

● LAYING ON OF HANDS

● HOLY COMMUNION

● ANOINTING WITH OIL

● PRAYER & PROPER MENTAL ATTITUDE

▯ ▯ ▯ ▯ ▯

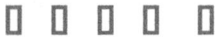

● THE WORD OF GOD

The Holy Bible says, "He sent his word, and healed them, and delivered them from their destructions." [Psalm 107:20.] God's Word heals: God's nature is healing, and he has given LIFE to his Word. You can be healed by knowing what God promises in his Word concerning healing. Find the promises God has made you in the Holy Bible for healing and for health, and then appropriate one or more of these promises for yourself.

Speak the promises of God to yourself (or to others). Your faith will rise as you do. "So then faith comes by hearing, and hearing by the Word of God." [Romans 10:17] As you confess (or speak aloud) the promises of God, your healing will come. Don't worry if you don't see it as soon as you think you should ... it has to happen!

Jesus taught that what you speak will come to pass if you believe it in your heart [Mark 11:23]. Don't talk sickness, or doubt, or unbelief anymore ... start talking healing, faith, and belief ... based upon what your Father God has promised you! Hearing and meditating upon God's Word help to produce healing, also. I have known people to be healed of conditions they have had for years by HEARING God's Word while I was preaching (both in worship services indoors and preaching outdoors).

"And they went forth, and preached everywhere, the Lord working with them, and confirming the word with signs following." [Mark 16:20]

Meditating (thinking deeply or fixing attention) upon God's Word brings life and health, also. Proverbs 4:20-22 tells us:

"My son, attend to my words; incline [or, direct] your ear unto my sayings. Let them not depart from your eyes; keep them in the middle of your heart. For they are LIFE unto those that find them, and HEALTH to all their flesh."

LAYING ON OF HANDS

After Messiah Jesus was raised from the dead and before he went back to Heaven, he said:

"And these signs shall follow them that believe; in my name shall they cast out devils; they shall speak

13

with new tongues ... they shall lay hands on the sick, and they shall recover." [Mark 16:17-18]

Notice three things Jesus told us:

- ▓ "In my name ..."
- ▓ " ... you shall lay hands on the sick,"
- ▓ " ... they [the sick] shall recover."

IN MY NAME - It is the name of **Jesus, the Messiah** ... the Holy One of God ... which is to accompany the laying on of hands. It is THE NAME that is above every name [Philippians 2:8-9]. The NAME of Jesus Christ joins God's power to your action.

The name of Jesus identifies you: it tells "sickness" and "demons" the authority behind your action and command; it tells them you belong to and are a believer in Jesus, the One who conquered them and their master, Satan! The name of Jesus identifies you with the One who CREATED the world and who BOUGHT IT BACK (after Adam's sin) with his own blood!

Use the name of Jesus with authority: as a citizen of Christ's kingdom. If you are in doubt, just whisper the name of Jesus for a while. "Jesus, Jesus, Jesus ...." It will call God's power to the scene! If it is a case of demon affliction, speak with authority (not your authority, but Christ's) and say: "You devil, come out! I command you in the name of Jesus Christ to come out of this person!"

14

YOU SHALL LAY HANDS ON THE SICK - If you are a believer in Jesus, then God wants to use you to heal others. You have the privilege, as well as the responsibility, of laying hands on the sick and praying for them: whether they are Christians or non-Christians. (See Luke 4:40; Acts 28:8.)

Your hands become Messiah's hands: his tools. The power of the Ruach HaKodesh (the Holy Spirit) flows through your hands. You may not see it, you may not feel it ... but it is POWER just the same. The devil is afraid of your touch! Because of distance, sometimes, you are not able to lay hands on the sick person. (The person you want to pray for may be in a different city.) You can then send them a "prayer cloth" to be laid on the body of the sick person.

"And God wrought special miracles by the hands of Paul: so that from his body were brought unto the sick handkerchiefs or aprons, and the diseases departed from them, and the evil spirits went out of them." [Acts 19:11-12]

Prayer cloths are very effective! Demons (evil spirits) are cast out, sick bodies are healed, minds are restored. Pray over the cloth (lay your hands on it) in the name of Jesus Christ and ask God to send deliverance, healing, and blessing. If you need a prayer cloth from Prince Handley, E-mail to:

princehandley@gmail.com
Make sure to include your postal mailing address.

If you are a Messianic Believer or a Christian, you have more POWER than the devil ever hoped to have! Satan is afraid of your handkerchief!!

THEY SHALL RECOVER - Forget what your mind or eyes tell you. Believe what God says. You may not see the person you pray for be healed as soon as you think you should ... however, you may see them be healed instantly. The important thing is to KNOW that they will recover. (In some cases the sick person may be hindering their healing; such cases will be covered later in this book under the section: "Prayer and Proper Mental Attitude".)

The Holy Spirit is God's agent on earth to supply the healing power of Christ. Whether the sick person is healed instantly or over a period of time - whether they feel God's power or not - Jesus promised, "These signs shall follow them that believe ... they shall lay hands on the sick, and they [the sick] shall recover." Your job is to serve **by faith** in obedience to Christ's command: "You go ... they shall recover." Read again Mark 16:15-18 and notice the command and the promise!

● PASSOVER AND HOLY COMMUNION

We should expect MIRACLES during either the Passover Seder or the Holy Communion (the Lord's Supper). We are celebrating what Messiah, the Lamb of God, did FOR US, and he told us to do this in order to remember him until he comes again.

16

"For as often as you eat this bread, and drink this cup, you SHOW the Lord's death until he comes [again]." [1 Corinthians 11:26]

The Holy Bible teaches us in 1 Corinthians 11:27-32 that we are to do two things when we come to the Lord's Supper:

Discern the Lord's body; and,

Examine ourselves.

To "discern" means to see his sacrifice for us as "distinct" from other things. See his body (the bread) beaten - even before the cross - as the Roman soldiers whip (or, flog) him, leaving his back bruised and striped with open wounds. See his head pierced by the crown of thorns, causing blood to flow down his face and chest. And then ... see his hands and feet nailed with rough spikes to the wooden cross. All of this **for us** ... and **for God**!

See his blood (the cup) shed for us: sinless blood, having good credit in the bank of Heaven. Not blood which inherited sin from Adam and his race, but **blood from a miracle birth** from above: as the Spirit of God breathed on the womb of a virgin, creating NEW LIFE from God. "In whom we have redemption THROUGH HIS BLOOD, the forgiveness of sins, according to the riches of his grace." [Ephesians 1:7]

Jesus' body and mind bore the punishment for **our** sins ... his blood paid the PRICE to redeem -- to

17

ransom -- **us**. And God raised him from the dead: Jesus is ALIVE to save and to heal you! Yes, miracles and healing are available in the Holy Communion by discerning the Lord's body ... seeing him and what he did for us.

He bore **our** sicknesses and diseases.

He carried (away) **our** pains.

He was wounded and bruised for **our** sin.

The LORD laid on him the sin of **us all**.

And with his stripes **WE ARE HEALED**!

ANOINTING WITH OIL

In the Holy Bible, anointing with oil is representative of the ministry of the Holy Spirit. Oil is a "type;" it represents the Holy Spirit. Carry a bottle of anointing oil with you at all times, ready for use. In James 5:14-15 we read:

"Is any sick among you? Let him call for the elders of the church; and let them pray over him, anointing him with oil in the name of the Lord.

And the prayer of faith shall save the sick, and the Lord shall raise him up; and if he has committed sins, they shall be forgiven him."

There is another type of anointing with oil which may be referred to as "evangelistic" anointing. It is just as much a part of evangelistic ministry as preaching, or teaching, or winning people to Christ. It does not require the sick person to "call" for the elders of the church; nor is it only for Christians. Mark 6:12-13 tells us:

"And they went out, and preached that men should repent. And they cast out many devils, and ANOINTED WITH OIL many that were sick, and healed them."

PRAYER AND PROPER MENTAL ATTITUDE

Your mind - and therefore your body - can be abused by many things. At times there are hindrances to healing: things or conditions that are causing the sickness or affliction, and that must be dealt with before healing can take place permanently. Things such as:

- Unforgiveness, bitterness, or resentment [Mark 11:25-26]
- Envy and strife [James 3:16]
- Improper food, rest, sunshine, or exercise [Isaiah 30:15]
- Speaking evil of, or causing harm to, God's ministers [1 Samuel 26:9]

- Involvement in the occult or in witchcraft [Deuteronomy 18:10-12]

- Association with religious cults [1 John 4:1-3 / 1 John 5:20]

Whether sickness is caused by disobeying God through an unforgiving spirit, strife, or resentment … involvement in the occult … or association with religious cults … Jesus Christ is the answer! **NOTE**: For help with deliverance, consult the book, *Healing Deliverance – Freedom from the Bondage of Satan*, by Prince Handley.

Through prayer we can come to God and ask him to **forgive** us of all these things; we can also ask him to **deliver** us, if necessary! 1 John 1:9 says, "If we confess our sins, he is faithful and just to forgive us our sins, and to cleanse us from all unrighteousness." In Psalm 50:15 we read, "Call upon me in the day of trouble: I will deliver you, and you shall glorify me."

Praise is also an important element in healing and is definitely inter-connected with prayer and proper mental attitude. Praise lets God know you believe **He will work** in your situation. Learn to lift your hands up to God and praise Him several times a day, at least for 30 seconds at a time.

- God lives in the praise of His people. *"But You are holy, O You that inhabits the praises of Israel."* (Psalm 22:3)

- The anointing breaks the yoke. Since God lives in the praise of His people, there is an anointing present with **true** praise, which can break an "assigned" attack on the body, mind or spirit. *"And it shall come to pass in that day, that **his burden shall be taken away from off thy shoulder, and his yoke from off thy neck**, and the yoke shall be destroyed because of the anointing."* (Isaiah 10:27)

- Praise brings victory. King Jehoshaphat and the inhabitants of Judah and Jerusalem won a large battle utilizing praise. (Read 2 Chronicles Chapter 20, verses 1-30 in the Tanakh.)

We see the importance of proper mental attitude in the life of Job. Job was afflicted by Satan with sore boils from his feet to his head. Also, the devil destroyed Job's wealth and killed his seven sons and three daughters. Job's experience was a rare, "once-in-the-Bible" case. It was allowed by God to prove that a certain man ("greatest of all the men in the east") would not curse God even if he lost everything, including his health.

It shows that Satan is a "destroyer," who causes sickness and disease. It shows that God is a "healer," and that God calls sickness "captivity." Job was a just man; even God said so. His experience presents a question that lots of people ask: "Why?"

Notice seven things:

1. Job's case was unique; it was NOT an example! Don't use it as an excuse to be sick.

2. Satan accused Job of serving God only because of God's blessing, protection and help.

3. Satan is the one, the Bible says, who STOLE Job's health, KILLED his children, and who DESTROYED his property. [Job, Chapters 1 and 2; John 10:10]

4. Job proved faithful in trial. Job did not sin with his lips or charge God foolishly. [Job 1:22 and 2:10]

5. The Bible calls Job's sickness and his loss -- "captivity." [Job 42:10]. Jesus said, "If the Son shall make you free, you shall be free indeed [John 8:36]

6. Job was healed! Because of proper mental attitude, Job prayed for his friends (who were not real friends); this was when God delivered Job. [Job 42:10]

7. "The Lord gave Job twice as much as he had before." "The Lord blessed the latter end of Job more than his beginning." [Job 42:10-12]

Even though Job lived on the other side of the cross (that is, before Christ) - not having the advantages of Christ's work and authority over Satan as we do - he was still healed through prayer and proper mental attitude. A **proper mental attitude** will cause you to have an instinctive reaction to sickness and ill-health: you will **refuse it** … knowing it does NOT belong to you!

You will speak to it, saying, "Sickness, I resist you in the name of Jesus Christ by whose stripes I am healed." Notice two things; you resisted the sickness by: 1) speaking to it; and, 2) using scripture (the Word of God).

The Holy Bible says in James 4:7, "Resist the devil, and he will flee from you." In Matthew 4:11, we see how Jesus resisted Satan. He did it the same way you are to do it: with the Word of God. Each time Jesus spoke to the devil, Jesus said, "It is written …"

Proper nutrition, rest, sunshine, and exercise are all beneficial to a proper mental attitude and maintenance of good health. Scriptural fasting and honoring the Lord's Day or Sabbath contribute, also, to a proper mental attitude; and are laws of God with built-in bonuses of health and blessing. Read Isaiah Chapter 58.

● CONCLUSION

It is God's will for you to be healed in every area of your life; and to maintain that healing: to walk in health! The most important thing to know is that you do not have to be sick. Jesus came to earth to heal. He took **your** sicknesses, **your** pains, **your** diseases ... and **your** sins ... on him, and with his stripes YOU ARE HEALED.

Jesus' body and mind took the punishment for your sins ... his sinless blood paid the price to buy you back to God. What Adam lost by disobedience, Jesus won back through obedience. Spiritual death ... which resulted in physical death, as well as sickness and disease ... was healed. The separation between man and God was ended for all who BELIEVE.

Now ... you can be healed. If you want to meet the Healer, Yeshua HaMashiach (Jesus, the Messiah), *NOW* is the time! Invite God's Son, Yeshua, to come into your life by praying this prayer:

➡ *"Lord Jesus, I know that you are The Great Physician. You loved me enough to shed your sinless blood and die for me on the cross that I might be healed. I know you are alive. Please forgive my sins, come into my life, and be my Master. Help me to live for you, and take me to Heaven when I die."*

If you prayed that prayer and meant it, then you have eternal life and your sins are ALL forgiven. You have been healed in your spirit. Know that God has heard and answered your prayer! The Bible says, "Whoever shall call upon the name of the Lord shall be saved." [Romans 10:13.] Notice, God did NOT say "may be saved" … "might be saved" … or even "probably," but his promise is: "Whoever shall call … SHALL BE saved!"

If you need physical or mental healing, pray and ask the Lord Jesus (Yeshua), the Son of God, to heal you … NOW! Or, obtain healing through any of the other methods God has made available:

- The Word of God

- Laying On of Hands

- Passover and Holy Communion

- Anointing with Oil

- Prayer and Proper Mental Attitude

Know that healing is yours because of:

- The PROMISES of God in his Word; and,

- The PROVISION of Christ in his Work for you!

☐ ☐ ☐ ☐ ☐

Now that you know YOUR RIGHT to divine healing and health, God wants you to share this "Good News" with others so they can be healed. Many times people find healing as they are helping others to be healed. It is a spiritual law that "what a man sows, that he also reaps."

If you have been blessed or received a miracle as a result of this booklet, E-mail us and let us know so we may rejoice! Email to:
universityofexcellence@gmail.com

BONUS: If you would like to subscribe to Prince Handley's **FREE** blog and teachings, which will give you helpful teaching plus prophecy as it pertains to current news events, E-mail to him at this address: **princehandley@gmail.com**. In the Subject line type the word "SUBSCRIBE."

As you lead others to the knowledge of healing and health through Messiah Jesus, you will be "sowing" for your own harvest of divine healing and health. Tell people about this booklet or share it with them.

God richly bless you!

"Freely you have received, freely give."

"How God anointed Yeshua (Jesus) of Nazareth with the Holy Spirit (Ruach HaKodesh) and with power, who went about doing good, and healing all that were oppressed of the devil; for God was with him."

Brit Chadashah (New Testament)
Acts 10:38

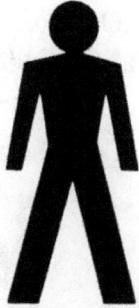

"You shall come to your grave in a full age, like a shock of corn comes in his season ...

We have searched it out and so it is; hear it and know it for your good."

Tanakh (Hebrew Scriptures)
Job 5:26-27

ᘔ ᘔ ᘔ

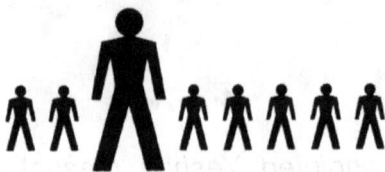

Prince Handley

Email prayer requests and praise reports to:
princehandley@gmail.com

Or write to:
Prince Handley
P.O. Box A
Downey, California 90241 USA

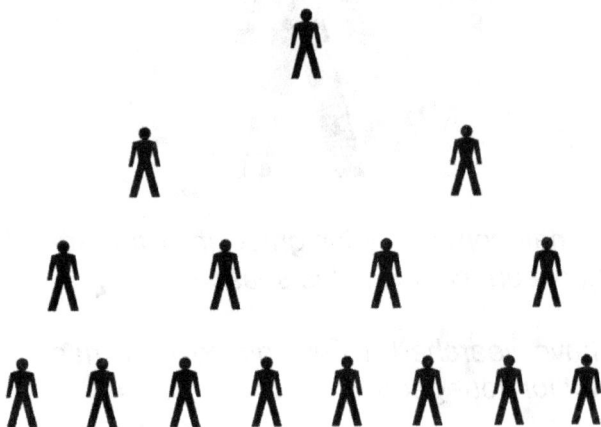

www.ingramcontent.com/pod-product-compliance
Lightning Source LLC
Chambersburg PA
CBHW060708280326
41933CB00012B/2348